Tourette Syndrome and Creativity

Exploring the Unique Gifts of TS Individuals.

Copyright Notice

Disclaimer

This book falls within the realm of nonfiction in the field of health. The information presented here is intended solely for general informational purposes and should not be considered a replacement for professional medical advice, diagnosis, or treatment. It is imperative to always seek guidance from a qualified healthcare provider or physician regarding any inquiries you may have about a medical condition. Please do not disregard professional medical advice or delay seeking it based on the content found in this book.

Contents

Introduction

In the intricate tapestry of human existence, there are countless threads that weave together to form the diverse and multifaceted mosaic of our world. Among these threads, some are more vibrant, more enigmatic, and more intriguing than others. Tourette Syndrome, a neurological condition characterized by involuntary vocalizations and repetitive movements, is one such thread. This book, "Tourette Syndrome and Creativity: Exploring the Unique Gifts of TS Individuals," embarks on a captivating journey through the lives of individuals who embody the dynamic interplay between neurological diversity and creativity.

Tourette Syndrome has long been viewed through a lens of stigma and misunderstanding, often overshadowing the remarkable abilities and extraordinary talents that can accompany it. Yet, beyond the tics and twitches, lies a hidden reservoir of creativity, innovation, and ingenuity that is often overlooked. The purpose of this book is to illuminate this hidden facet, to celebrate the remarkable gifts of those who live with Tourette Syndrome, and to shed light on the astonishing fusion of neurodiversity and creativity.

As we delve into the pages of this book, we will meet individuals who have harnessed their unique neurological wiring to achieve extraordinary feats in different domains. We will explore the fascinating connection between Tourette Syndrome and creativity, understanding how the very traits that manifest as tics and compulsions can also serve as a wellspring of inspiration and innovation.

"Tourette Syndrome and Creativity" is a testament to the resilience and resourcefulness of those who dare to defy expectations. Through personal stories, expert insights, and a deep dive into the science behind Tourette Syndrome, we aim to redefine the narrative surrounding this condition, casting it in a new, compassionate, and more accurate light. By the end of this journey, we hope to foster a greater appreciation for the distinctive talents and invaluable contributions of TS individuals.

Join me on this voyage of discovery, one that uncovers the remarkable and often overlooked gifts of individuals living with Tourette Syndrome. Together, let us celebrate the extraordinary creativity that resides within the unique tapestry of TS minds and explore the profound impact it has had on our world.

Chapter 1

Understanding Tourette Syndrome

Tourette Syndrome (TS) is a complex neurological disorder that has fascinated researchers, clinicians, and the general public for decades. It is a condition characterized by involuntary motor and vocal tics, which can range from subtle and barely noticeable to severe and disruptive. While TS has long been associated with its distinct motor and vocal symptoms, it has also been linked to a range of cognitive and emotional challenges. However, this intriguing condition is not just defined by its challenges; it has also been associated with remarkable strengths, particularly in the realm of creativity.

The Nature of Tics and Their Impact

Tics are the hallmark of Tourette Syndrome. They are sudden, rapid, and involuntary movements or vocalizations that often appear with little or no preceding urge. Tics can be categorized into two main types:

- **Motor Tics**: These involve involuntary movements of the body. Common motor tics include eye blinking, head jerking, shoulder shrugging, facial grimacing, and more complex motor tics like touching, hopping, or gesturing. Motor tics can be subtle or pronounced, ranging from barely noticeable to highly disruptive.

- **Vocal Tics**: Vocal tics entail involuntary vocal sounds or utterances. These may include throat clearing, grunting, sniffing, or more complex vocalizations such as the repetition of words or phrases. Some individuals with TS may exhibit coprolalia, which involves involuntary and socially inappropriate swearing or obscene language, but this is a relatively rare symptom.

Tourette Syndrome is considered a spectrum disorder, which means that the severity and types of tics vary widely among individuals. Tics tend to emerge in childhood, typically between the ages of 5 and 10, and often peak during the teenage years. Over time, tics may change in type, frequency, and intensity. Some individuals experience transient tics that disappear in adulthood, while others continue to have tics throughout their lives.

The impact of TS on an individual's life can be significant. Tics can be physically and emotionally distressing, leading to discomfort and challenges in various settings, including school, work, and social situations. The social stigma associated with tics can also contribute to feelings of isolation and low self-esteem.

Co-occurring Conditions and Challenges

Tourette Syndrome is often accompanied by a range of co-occurring conditions and challenges, which can vary from person to person. Some common co-occurring conditions include:

Attention Deficit Hyperactivity Disorder (ADHD): The concurrent presence of Tourette Syndrome (TS) and Attention-Deficit/Hyperactivity Disorder (ADHD) is not uncommon. These are two distinct neurodevelopmental conditions that can co-occur in some individuals, and understanding their relationship is essential for effective diagnosis and management.

Attention-Deficit/Hyperactivity Disorder (ADHD) is another neurodevelopmental condition, characterized by difficulties with attention, impulse control, and hyperactivity. ADHD can manifest in different ways, with three main subtypes: inattentive type, hyperactive-impulsive type, and combined type.

There is a notable co-occurrence of TS and ADHD. Research suggests that approximately 50% of individuals with TS also experience symptoms of ADHD. This high overlap has prompted further exploration of the relationship between the two conditions.

Some studies suggest that there may be shared neurobiological mechanisms between TS and ADHD. Dysregulation of certain neurotransmitters, such as dopamine, is implicated in both conditions.

Both TS and ADHD may present with overlapping symptoms, such as inattention and impulsivity. This can complicate the diagnostic process, as these shared features may make it challenging to differentiate between the two conditions.

Children and adolescents with concurrent TS and ADHD may face difficulties in school. Inattention and impulsivity can affect academic performance, and the presence of tics may add to the challenges, especially if they are disruptive in the classroom.

The co-occurrence of TS and ADHD can lead to social challenges. TS individuals may experience teasing or social difficulties due to their tics, while ADHD-related impulsivity can impact relationships.

Obsessive-Compulsive Disorder (OCD): The co-occurrence of Tourette Syndrome (TS) and Obsessive-Compulsive Disorder (OCD) is a well-documented phenomenon. Both TS and OCD are neurodevelopmental conditions that share some similarities and can manifest concurrently in some individuals. Understanding this concurrent presentation is essential for accurate diagnosis and effective management.

Obsessive-Compulsive Disorder (OCD) is characterized by the presence of obsessions and compulsions. Obsessions are intrusive, unwanted, and distressing thoughts, images, or urges, while compulsions are repetitive behaviors or mental acts that an individual feels compelled to perform to alleviate distress.

TS and OCD are known to co-occur more frequently than expected by chance. Studies have reported that approximately 20-30% of individuals with TS also have comorbid OCD.

There are some similarities in symptoms between TS and OCD. Tics can be seen as a form of compulsive behavior, as individuals with TS may experience an irresistible urge to perform the tics, similar to the compulsion seen in OCD.

Both TS and OCD are believed to involve disruptions in the basal ganglia and dopaminergic pathways in the brain. This shared neurobiology may contribute to the concurrent presentation of these conditions in some individuals.

The co-occurrence of TS and OCD can lead to compounded symptoms, potentially increasing distress and functional impairment. For example, individuals may experience tics related to their obsessions or compulsions.

Diagnosing TS and OCD concurrently can be complex because of symptom overlap and shared features. Clinicians need to carefully differentiate between the two conditions to develop an appropriate treatment plan.

Anxiety and Depression: The co-occurrence of Tourette Syndrome (TS) and anxiety or depression is not uncommon. Individuals with TS often face a range of challenges, including social stigma, tic-related distress, and difficulty coping with the symptoms of the condition. These challenges can contribute to the development of anxiety and depression.

Anxiety disorders commonly co-occur with TS. Generalized Anxiety Disorder, Social Anxiety Disorder, and Specific Phobias are examples of anxiety disorders that may manifest in individuals with TS. Anxiety can result from the stress and uncertainty associated with tics, as well as the social challenges and stigma that TS individuals may encounter.

Depression is another condition that can co-occur with TS. Individuals with TS may experience depressive symptoms due to the distress caused by tics, difficulties in social interactions, or feelings of isolation and alienation.

Research has shown a higher prevalence of anxiety and depression in individuals with TS compared to the general population. The challenges posed by TS can contribute to the development of these conditions.

Anxiety and depression can share symptoms with TS, making it challenging to distinguish between the conditions. For example, the frustration and distress associated with tics can be mistaken for symptoms of anxiety or depression.

The co-occurrence of TS with anxiety and depression can exacerbate distress. Managing the symptoms of all three conditions can be overwhelming and negatively impact an individual's quality of life.

Anxiety and depression may lead individuals to withdraw from social interactions, increasing feelings of isolation. This can further affect their mental health and overall well-being.

Learning Disabilities: Some individuals with TS may also have specific learning disabilities that can impact their academic performance. These may include difficulties with reading, writing, or math.

Social Challenges: The tics associated with TS can lead to social challenges, as individuals may be teased, bullied, or face social exclusion. Coprolalia, in particular, can be socially isolating.

Health and Safety Concerns: Certain tics, especially those involving physical movements, can pose safety risks, such as accidentally injuring oneself or others.

Quality of Life: TS can affect an individual's overall quality of life, as it may require ongoing medical care, therapy, and support to manage symptoms and challenges effectively.

Understanding Tourette Syndrome requires recognition of its diverse presentation and its potential impact on various aspects of an individual's life. The condition is not solely defined by tics but involves a complex interplay of co-occurring conditions and challenges. Successful management often involves a multidisciplinary approach, including medical, psychological, and educational support, to help individuals with TS navigate the complexities of the condition and enhance their quality of life.

Chapter 2

Tourette Syndrome (TS) and Age

The severity of Tourette Syndrome (TS) can vary from person to person and often changes over time. While the condition typically emerges in childhood, its impact can evolve as individuals with TS progress through various life stages. Here's an overview of how the severity of TS can change with age:

Childhood Onset: TS typically begins in childhood, often between the ages of 5 and 10. In many cases, the initial tics that appear are simple motor tics, like eye blinking or head jerking. The severity during childhood can range from mild to moderate, with tics often occurring sporadically and not significantly interfering with daily activities.

Adolescence: Adolescence is a period of transition in terms of the severity of TS. Tics may become more noticeable and complex during these years. Social challenges can arise as teenagers become more self-aware and may feel embarrassed or isolated due to their tics. Stressors like academic demands and peer interactions can exacerbate tic severity.

Adulthood: For many individuals with TS, the severity of tics decreases as they move into adulthood. As people mature, they often develop better strategies for managing their tics, including finding ways to suppress them or release the urge without the observable tic. Although tics may still be present, they may become less frequent, less noticeable, or milder in adulthood.

Elderly Age: In many cases, tics tend to further decline in severity in older age. As individuals age, they often experience a reduction in the intensity and frequency of tics, and some may even see their tics disappear entirely. Factors such as life experience, self-acceptance, and the development of coping mechanisms contribute to the milder nature of tics in older individuals.

The severity of Tourette Syndrome can vary throughout an individual's life. While tics often become less severe as people move into adulthood and beyond, the experience of TS is highly individual. Support, understanding, and appropriate interventions can play a crucial role in helping individuals manage their tics and navigate the evolving nature of their condition.

It's important to note that TS is highly variable, and not everyone follows the same trajectory. Some individuals may continue to experience moderate to severe tics throughout their lives, while others may have mild or even transient tics. Co-occurring conditions, such as ADHD or OCD, can also influence the severity and progression of TS.

Chapter 3

Tourette Syndrome (TS) and Stress

Stress is a well-recognized trigger for tics in individuals with Tourette Syndrome (TS). While the exact mechanisms are not fully understood, it is believed that the relationship between stress and tics is complex and involves various physiological and psychological factors. Here's how stress can trigger or exacerbate tics in people with TS:

1. **Increased Neurological Sensitivity:** Stress activates the body's "fight or flight" response, which involves the release of stress hormones like cortisol and adrenaline. In individuals with TS, this

heightened state of arousal can make them more sensitive to sensory and emotional stimuli, potentially increasing the likelihood of tics.

2. **Anticipatory Anxiety:** The anticipation of stressful events or situations, often referred to as "anticipatory anxiety," can trigger tics. Individuals with TS may become anxious about the possibility of tics occurring in public or during important events, leading to an increase in tic frequency.

3. **Tension and Muscle Contraction:** Stress can lead to muscle tension and increased muscle contractions. For individuals with TS who experience motor tics, stress may exacerbate these symptoms by increasing

muscle tension, making it more challenging to suppress or control tics.

4. **Emotional Response:** The emotional response to stress, such as frustration, anxiety, or anger, can trigger or worsen tics. Emotional stressors can activate the neural pathways associated with tics, leading to their expression.

5. **Social and Performance Anxiety:** Stress related to social interactions, such as giving presentations or attending social gatherings, can be a significant trigger for tics. The fear of judgment or the pressure to conform to social norms can increase tic frequency.

6. **Co-Occurring Conditions:** Many individuals with TS also have co-occurring conditions like anxiety disorders or Attention-Deficit/Hyperactivity Disorder (ADHD). These conditions can heighten overall stress levels and, in turn, exacerbate tics.

7. **Cognitive Factors:** Stress can interfere with cognitive processes, making it more challenging for individuals with TS to suppress tics consciously. The cognitive effort required to inhibit tics can become less effective during stressful moments.

Managing Stress to Reduce Tic Severity

Managing stress is a key aspect of helping individuals with TS reduce the severity of their tics. Strategies for stress management include:

1. **Cognitive-Behavioral Therapy (CBT):** CBT can help individuals with TS identify and manage stressors and develop coping mechanisms to deal with anticipatory anxiety and emotional responses to stress.

2. **Relaxation Techniques:** Techniques such as deep breathing, meditation, and progressive muscle relaxation can help reduce overall stress levels and improve the ability to manage tics.

3. **Exercise:** Regular physical activity can be an effective way to reduce stress and improve overall well-being. It may also help decrease the frequency and intensity of tics.

4. **Support Systems:** A strong support system of family and friends who understand and provide emotional support can help individuals with TS manage stress more effectively.

5. **Medication:** In some cases, healthcare professionals may prescribe medications to help manage the symptoms of TS and reduce the impact of tics during periods of heightened stress.

While the exact mechanisms are not entirely clear, it is well-established that stress can trigger or exacerbate tics in individuals with Tourette Syndrome. Stress management strategies, in combination with therapy and social support, are crucial in helping individuals with TS reduce the impact of stress on their tics and overall quality of life.

Chapter 4

Unravelling the TS-Creativity Connection

Understanding the intricate relationship between Tourette Syndrome (TS) and creativity is a multifaceted endeavor. This connection has captivated the interest of scholars and researchers for years, and it is comprised of both historical perspectives and contemporary scientific investigations. In this section, we will delve into the TS-creativity connection, examining its historical roots and the current research findings that shed light on this fascinating phenomenon.

Historical Perspectives and Case Studies

Historical accounts of individuals with TS who exhibited extraordinary creativity offer a compelling starting point for exploring the TS-creativity connection. Several notable figures throughout history have been posthumously diagnosed or speculated to have had TS based on their documented behaviors. These individuals often exemplify how TS might intersect with exceptional talents:

Samuel Johnson

Samuel Johnson, an 18th-century literary giant, was a man of extraordinary intellectual prowess. His contribution to the English language, through his monumental work "A Dictionary of the English Language," remains unparalleled. Yet, behind the brilliant wordsmith was a man who grappled with a neurological condition that would later be recognized as Tourette Syndrome (TS).

Early Life and Symptoms: Samuel Johnson was born in Lichfield, Staffordshire, England, on September 18, 1709. From an early age, he displayed a host of unusual and repetitive behaviors, both in terms of motor and vocal tics. His tics included blinking his eyes incessantly, making involuntary grimaces, and emitting various throat-clearing sounds.

Social Stigma and Misunderstanding: In Johnson's time, little was known about TS, and there were no established medical explanations for these symptoms. People around him were often perplexed and ignorant of the nature of his condition, which caused Johnson considerable social isolation and ridicule. He was frequently described as awkward, strange, or even mad, leading to a sense of alienation and difficulty forming social relationships.

Despite these challenges, Johnson possessed a relentless and curious intellect, seeking solace in books and the pursuit of knowledge. He was a voracious reader and developed a deep love for the written word, setting the stage for his future contributions to English literature.

Creative Triumph Over Adversity: Ironically, Johnson's TS, while causing him great discomfort and social hardship, may have played a significant role in shaping his literary and intellectual genius. His condition seemed to have fueled his penchant for meticulousness and precision in his work. The painstaking task of compiling the dictionary, which he undertook single-handedly, demonstrates an extraordinary attention to detail.

"A Dictionary of the English Language," published in 1755, was a groundbreaking achievement that laid the foundation for the modern English lexicon. It was not merely a compilation of words and their meanings but a work of immense scholarship and a testament to Johnson's formidable intellect.

Legacy: Samuel Johnson's legacy extends far beyond the pages of the dictionary. His literary and critical works, such as "The Lives of the English Poets" and "Rasselas," continue to be studied and revered today. His mastery of the English language and his contribution to its standardization have left an indelible mark on the world of letters.

In retrospect, Samuel Johnson's struggle with TS serves as a poignant reminder of the resilience and creativity that can emerge from adversity. Despite the challenges posed by his neurological condition, Johnson's commitment to intellectual pursuits and his contributions to literature have left an enduring legacy. He stands as a testament to the human spirit's capacity to triumph over physical and social obstacles, leaving a remarkable imprint on the world of words and ideas.

Dr. Samuel Taylor Johnson

Dr. Samuel Taylor Johnson, an American neurologist born in 1831, holds a significant place in the history of medical science for his pioneering work in the field of neurology. Dr. Johnson's research and clinical observations were instrumental in the early understanding and recognition of Tourette Syndrome (TS), a neurological condition characterized by repetitive, involuntary movements and vocalizations known as tics.

Early Life and Career: Born in the United States during the 19th century, Dr. Samuel T. Johnson embarked on a medical career during a time when the medical understanding of neurological conditions was still in its infancy. Throughout his medical training and subsequent practice, Dr. Johnson began to notice certain patterns and behaviors in his patients that didn't fit into the existing diagnostic categories of the time.

Recognition of Tourette Syndrome: Dr. Johnson's keen observations and meticulous record-keeping led to the identification of a distinct set of symptoms that were consistently recurring among some of his patients. He noticed that some individuals exhibited involuntary motor tics, such as blinking, grimacing, or sudden jerking movements, along with vocal tics, including throat-clearing or grunting sounds. This cluster of symptoms, which he initially referred to as "involuntary impulsive tics," laid the foundation for the recognition of Tourette Syndrome.

Publication and Legacy: In 1885, Dr. Samuel T. Johnson published a comprehensive clinical account of the condition he had observed in a medical journal, which marked the first formal description of what we now know as Tourette Syndrome. His work shed light on the disorder, providing medical professionals with a basis for understanding and diagnosing TS in the years to come.

While his contributions were instrumental in recognizing and defining the condition, Dr. Johnson's findings were largely overlooked during his lifetime. It wasn't until the 20th century that Tourette Syndrome gained more widespread recognition and research attention. Today, Dr. Samuel T. Johnson is remembered as a pioneer in the field of neurology and for his pivotal role in the early understanding of TS.

Dr. Samuel T. Johnson's legacy is deeply intertwined with the history of Tourette Syndrome. His meticulous clinical observations and determination to document and understand the condition paved the way for future generations of researchers and clinicians to delve deeper into TS and provide support and treatment for those affected by it. Dr. Johnson's dedication to his patients and his contribution to medical knowledge have left an indelible mark on the field of neurology and continue to benefit those who live with Tourette Syndrome.

Jim Eisenreich

Jim Eisenreich, born on April 18, 1959, is a remarkable figure in the world of sports who overcame significant challenges associated with Tourette Syndrome (TS) to become a successful Major League Baseball (MLB) player. His story is a testament to perseverance, determination, and the ability to excel in the face of adversity.

Early Struggles: Eisenreich's journey with TS began in his early years when he began to display the characteristic tics and involuntary movements associated with the condition. As a child, he experienced social isolation and bullying due to his tics, making him an easy target for ridicule. Despite these challenges, Eisenreich's love for baseball began to blossom, and he used the sport as an outlet to express himself and find solace.

Professional Career: Eisenreich's talent on the baseball field was evident from a young age. His dedication and hard work led him to be drafted by the Minnesota Twins in the

16th round of the 1980 MLB draft. He made his MLB debut with the Twins in 1982, and it was during his time in the league that he became more open about his struggle with TS.

Overcoming Challenges: Throughout his career, Jim Eisenreich continued to battle the tics and twitches associated with TS, even on the baseball field. However, he did not let this neurological condition hinder his performance. Instead, he used his experiences to raise awareness and provide inspiration to others facing similar challenges.

Eisenreich went on to play for several MLB teams, including the Kansas City Royals, Philadelphia Phillies, and Florida Marlins. His consistency at the plate and his ability to play multiple positions made him a valuable asset to his teams. In 1997, he was a key player for the Florida Marlins, helping the team win the World Series.

Advocacy and Legacy: Jim Eisenreich's openness about his TS and his ability to succeed in professional sports inspired many individuals living with neurological conditions. He became a dedicated advocate, using his platform to raise awareness about TS and other neurological disorders. Eisenreich founded the Jim Eisenreich Foundation for Children with Tourette Syndrome, which aimed to support children facing neurological challenges and to enhance their quality of life.

In recognition of his contributions to both the world of baseball and his advocacy efforts, Jim Eisenreich is celebrated as a remarkable figure who demonstrated that with perseverance, determination, and support, individuals with TS can achieve their dreams. His story serves as a source of inspiration for many, both in the field of sports and in the broader context of life's challenges and triumphs.

Pete Davidson

Pete Davidson, born on November 16, 1993, is a popular American comedian, actor, and writer known for his sharp wit and self-deprecating humor. He's also one of the few public figures who have openly discussed their experience with Tourette Syndrome (TS), shedding light on the condition and challenging stigmas surrounding it.

Early Life and Diagnosis: Pete Davidson was diagnosed with Tourette Syndrome at a young age, which made his childhood and adolescent years a unique and sometimes challenging experience.

Embracing Comedy: Davidson's path to comedy began at an early age, and he turned to humor as a way to cope with the challenges of TS. He found solace in making people laugh, and his genuine and self-aware style resonated with audiences.

In 2014, Davidson joined the cast of "Saturday Night Live" (SNL), becoming one of the youngest cast members in the show's history. His appearances on SNL and his stand-up comedy routines often incorporate his experiences with TS and other personal struggles, offering a humorous and candid perspective on living with a neurological condition.

Advocacy and Awareness: Pete Davidson's openness about his TS has been instrumental in raising awareness about the condition and challenging misconceptions. He has used his platform to educate the public about the realities of TS, emphasizing that it is not just about tics but also involves other challenges, such as social stigmatization and associated mental health issues like anxiety and depression.

By sharing his journey and using humor to address sensitive topics, Davidson has inspired others with TS to embrace their differences and pursue their passions. He has shown that individuals with TS can excel in various fields and lead fulfilling lives.

Challenges and Triumphs: While Davidson's career has been marked by numerous successes, he continues to face the challenges associated with TS. The unpredictability of tics can be particularly challenging for someone in the public eye, but Davidson's resilience and determination have allowed him to continue performing and making people laugh.

In addition to his comedy career, Davidson has also pursued acting and has appeared in films and television series, further expanding his creative reach.

In conclusion, Pete Davidson's journey from a young boy diagnosed with Tourette Syndrome to a successful comedian and actor is a testament to his talent, resilience, and ability to use humor to connect with audiences. His openness about TS has played a pivotal role in increasing understanding and acceptance of the condition, inspiring others to embrace their uniqueness, and showing that even in the face of challenges, one can thrive and succeed in the world of entertainment and beyond.

Michael Wolff

Michael Wolff, born on July 31, 1952, is an accomplished American jazz pianist, bandleader, composer, and actor. He is known for his remarkable contributions to the world of music and his resilience in the face of a neurological challenge: Tourette Syndrome (TS).

Early Life and Diagnosis: Michael Wolff's journey began in Victorville, California. His love for music and his natural talent for the piano became evident at a young age. However, it was also during his childhood that he was diagnosed with TS, a neurological condition characterized by repetitive, involuntary movements and vocalizations known as tics.

The Challenges of TS: Tourette Syndrome presented numerous challenges for Wolff, as the condition often comes with tics that can be distracting, both to the individual experiencing them and to those around them. Wolff's tics included facial grimaces, head jerking, and vocal tics, which could have disrupted his musical performances and daily life.

Resilience and Music: Despite the challenges posed by TS, Michael Wolff's passion for music was unwavering. He used the piano as an outlet to express himself, and the act of playing allowed him to temporarily suppress his tics. Wolff's extraordinary musical abilities shone through even in the face of this neurological condition.

Success and Recognition: Wolff's career took off when he began performing in New York City in the late 1970s. He became a well-respected jazz pianist, known for his dynamic and energetic performances. He recorded numerous albums and led his own bands, earning a dedicated following in the jazz world.

Television and Acting: In addition to his music career, Michael Wolff became widely recognized for his role as the bandleader on "The Arsenio Hall Show" during the late 1980s and early 1990s. His television appearances allowed him to reach a broader audience and further showcase his musical talents.

TS Advocacy: Throughout his life, Wolff has been open about his experiences with TS and the impact it has had on his life and career. He has used his platform to advocate for awareness and understanding of the condition, breaking down stereotypes and stigma associated with TS.

Dash Mihok

Dash Mihok, born on May 24, 1974, is a well-regarded American actor known for his versatile performances in film, television, and theater. What makes Dash Mihok's journey particularly remarkable is that he has achieved acclaim in the entertainment industry while living with Tourette Syndrome (TS).

Early Life and Diagnosis: Dash Mihok's life took an unusual turn when, as a child, he was diagnosed with TS. This condition often presents a range of motor tics (such as eye blinking, head jerking, and facial grimacing) and vocal tics (including throat-clearing and grunting sounds). For a budding actor, such symptoms might have seemed like a significant obstacle, but Mihok refused to let TS dictate the course of his life.

Passion for Acting: From a young age, Dash Mihok displayed a deep passion for acting. It was an interest he pursued tirelessly, using his love for the craft as a way to cope with the challenges posed by TS. Through acting, he found an outlet for creative expression and a means to channel his emotions.

Early Career and Resilience: Mihok's determination to succeed as an actor eventually led him to New York City, where he honed his craft and overcame the challenges posed by TS. His early career was marked by persistence, as he diligently worked in theater productions, building a foundation of experience and expertise that would later serve him well in Hollywood.

Breakthrough Roles: Dash Mihok's breakthrough came with his appearance in the critically acclaimed film "The Thin Red Line" (1998), directed by Terrence Malick. His performance in this war epic, alongside a star-studded cast, garnered attention and praise for its depth and authenticity.

Notable Work: Mihok's acting career continued to flourish as he took on various roles in both film and television. He is perhaps best known for his portrayal of Bunchy Donovan in the television series "Ray Donovan." His performance in this role was praised for its emotional depth and the authentic portrayal of a character who, like Mihok himself, grapples with TS.

Advocacy and Awareness: Dash Mihok has used his platform and personal experiences to raise awareness about Tourette Syndrome. He has been a strong advocate for those living with the condition, emphasizing the importance of acceptance, understanding, and support.

Dash Mihok's journey is a testament to the power of passion and determination. Despite living with TS, he has carved out a successful career in the entertainment industry, showcasing his talent as an actor and using his experiences to advocate for those facing similar challenges. His resilience and the authenticity he brings to his roles have earned him both respect and admiration in the world of acting. Dash Mihok's story serves as an inspiration for all those striving to overcome obstacles and pursue their dreams, no matter the odds.

Tim Howard

Tim Howard, born on March 6, 1979, is a legendary American soccer goalkeeper who has earned recognition and respect both in the United States and internationally for his exceptional talent, dedication, and sportsmanship. What makes Tim Howard's story even more inspiring is his open discussion about living with Tourette Syndrome (TS).

Early Life and Diagnosis: Tim Howard's journey began in North Brunswick, New Jersey, where he was diagnosed with TS at the age of nine. The condition manifested through tics such as facial grimacing and eye blinking, which could be distracting and challenging for a budding soccer player.

However, Howard's family and coaches provided unwavering support, encouraging his passion for the sport.

Soccer as an Outlet: Soccer became more than just a sport for Tim Howard; it became an outlet for his energy and emotions. Playing between the goalposts offered him a unique way to channel his focus and provided relief from the symptoms of TS. He learned to suppress his tics during matches, allowing his talent and dedication to shine through.

Early Career and Resilience: Howard's career took off when he signed with the North Jersey Imperials and then with the MetroStars (now known as the New York Red Bulls) in Major League Soccer (MLS).

His strong performances and resilience in the face of TS caught the attention of soccer enthusiasts and professionals alike.

Notable Achievements: Tim Howard's career reached new heights when he moved to the English Premier League (EPL) in 2003, signing with Manchester United. He subsequently played for Everton, where he became a fan favorite and established himself as one of the best goalkeepers in the league. Howard's exceptional shot-stopping abilities and leadership on the field earned him numerous accolades and records.

Memorable World Cup Performance: One of the defining moments of Howard's career came during the 2014 FIFA World Cup. As the starting goalkeeper for the United States, he put on an extraordinary performance against Belgium in the round of 16, making a record-breaking 16 saves in a single World Cup match. This heroic effort endeared him to fans around the world and led to the coining of the term "Tim Howard-ing."

Advocacy and Awareness: Tim Howard has used his position as a soccer icon to raise awareness about Tourette Syndrome. He has been a vocal advocate for individuals living with TS, emphasizing the importance of acceptance, understanding, and support for those facing neurological conditions.

These famous creatives demonstrate that TS can coexist with exceptional talents and creative pursuits. Their stories not only raise awareness about the condition but also emphasize the importance of embracing one's uniqueness and leveraging it to create art, music, comedy, and other forms of creative expression.

The creative minds of individuals with Tourette Syndrome are a testament to the human capacity to turn challenges into opportunities for self-expression and achievement. Personal stories and famous figures with TS offer powerful examples of how creativity can thrive in the presence of this complex neurological condition, reminding us that the human spirit is resilient, diverse, and endlessly creative.

Chapter 5

Current Research and Findings

Contemporary research into the TS-creativity connection has yielded a more nuanced and evidence-based understanding. Although definitive conclusions remain elusive, several studies have explored the potential mechanisms and correlations:

Cognitive Flexibility

Cognitive flexibility is a crucial aspect of the relationship between Tourette Syndrome (TS) and creativity. Cognitive flexibility refers to the ability to adapt one's thinking and approach to various situations, tasks, and challenges. In the context of the TS-creativity relationship, cognitive flexibility can play a significant role in fostering creative thinking. Here's how it works:

1. **Thinking Outside the Box:** Individuals with TS often exhibit cognitive flexibility, which allows them to think outside the box. They are more inclined to consider alternative solutions and approaches to problems, leading to creative thinking. Their ability to break away from conventional thought patterns can result in innovative and unconventional ideas.

2. **Adaptation to Change:** Cognitive flexibility enables individuals to adapt quickly to changes and uncertainty. In the creative process, change and uncertainty

are common, and individuals with TS may be better equipped to embrace and navigate these challenges, ultimately leading to creative problem-solving and adaptability.

3. **Multidimensional Thinking:** TS may encourage individuals to engage in multidimensional thinking, where they can consider a wide range of factors and variables simultaneously. This holistic approach to problem-solving and creativity allows for a deeper exploration of ideas and concepts.

4. **Synthesizing Information:** Cognitive flexibility is closely associated with the ability to synthesize information from various sources and apply it to creative

endeavors. Individuals with TS may excel at synthesizing seemingly unrelated information to create novel and unique works.

5. **Improvisation:** Many creative fields, such as music and art, involve a level of improvisation. Individuals with TS may thrive in such environments due to their cognitive flexibility, allowing them to adapt and improvise more effectively.

6. **Embracing Uncertainty:** Creative endeavors often involve dealing with ambiguity and uncertainty. TS individuals' cognitive flexibility may make them more comfortable with these aspects of the creative process, enabling them to explore new ideas and possibilities.

7. **Problem-Solving:** Creative thinking frequently requires effective problem-solving. Cognitive flexibility helps individuals approach problems from different angles and find creative solutions. The TS-creativity relationship is strengthened when individuals with TS apply this flexible problem-solving approach to their creative work.

Cognitive flexibility in individuals with Tourette Syndrome can foster creative thinking by encouraging unconventional approaches, adaptability to change, and a holistic perspective. This flexibility in thought processes contributes to the development of innovative and unique ideas and creative solutions in various fields.

Divergent Thinking:

Divergent thinking plays a significant role in the relationship between Tourette Syndrome (TS) and creativity. Divergent thinking is a cognitive process characterized by the ability to generate multiple unique and creative solutions to a given problem. Here's how divergent thinking may be related to creativity in individuals with TS:

1. **Enhanced Cognitive Flexibility:** Divergent thinking is closely linked to cognitive flexibility—the ability to shift between different perspectives and ideas. Some individuals with TS exhibit an increased level of cognitive flexibility, which can be beneficial for creative thinking. They may find it easier to break away from

conventional thought patterns and explore a wide range of possibilities when problem-solving or engaging in creative activities.

2. **Novel Idea Generation:** Divergent thinking encourages the generation of novel and unique ideas. Individuals with TS may excel in this aspect as their neurological condition often leads to unconventional thought patterns. They may come up with unexpected, fresh, and innovative solutions to problems or creative challenges, which is a hallmark of creativity.

3. **Reduced Inhibition:** TS is associated with difficulties in inhibiting certain behaviors, such as tics. Paradoxically, this reduced

ability to inhibit thoughts and actions might actually be advantageous for creativity. It can lower the barriers to unconventional thinking, allowing individuals with TS to explore ideas that others might dismiss or overlook.

4. **Tolerance for Ambiguity:** Divergent thinking often requires a tolerance for ambiguity, as creative processes can be messy and uncertain. Individuals with TS may be more comfortable with ambiguity and chaos in their creative work, as their neurological condition has already introduced unpredictability into their lives.

5. **Interconnected Ideas:** The tics and repetitive behaviors associated with TS sometimes reveal interconnected ideas or patterns. Some individuals with TS have reported that their tics are linked to certain mental images or associations. This mental linkage between ideas can be harnessed for creative inspiration, helping them to draw connections between seemingly unrelated concepts.

6. **Unconventional Solutions:** Creativity often thrives on unconventional, out-of-the-box thinking. TS can lead individuals to view problems and challenges from unique angles, allowing them to develop unconventional solutions that set their creative work apart from the norm.

The relationship between divergent thinking and creativity in individuals with Tourette Syndrome is a potential benefit of the condition. It can foster unconventional thinking, increased cognitive flexibility, and the generation of novel ideas, all of which contribute to a unique approach to creative problem-solving and artistic expression.

Obsessive-Compulsive Traits

The relationship between Obsessive-Compulsive Traits (OCTs) and creativity in individuals with Tourette Syndrome (TS) is a complex and multifaceted one. Obsessive-Compulsive Traits refer to the presence of obsessive or compulsive tendencies without necessarily meeting the full diagnostic criteria for Obsessive-Compulsive Disorder (OCD). Here's how these traits may be linked to creativity in individuals with TS:

1. **Enhanced Attention to Detail:** Some individuals with TS and OCTs may have an enhanced ability to focus on minute details, which can be a valuable asset in creative endeavors. This heightened attention to detail allows them to notice things that others might overlook, contributing to a richer and more intricate creative output.

2. **Persistence and Perseverance:** Individuals with OCTs often exhibit a strong drive to repeat certain behaviors or thoughts. This persistence and perseverance can be channeled into

creative pursuits, as they are less likely to give up when facing challenges or obstacles in the creative process. The ability to continually refine and improve one's work is essential for artistic or intellectual success.

3. **Idea Generation:** TS individuals with OCTs might engage in obsessive thinking patterns, continually generating and refining ideas. While these obsessive thoughts may be unrelated to their creative pursuits, some of these ideas could serendipitously lead to creative breakthroughs in their work.

4. **Unconventional Thinking:** Creativity often thrives on unconventional thinking. Individuals with TS and OCTs may have a

propensity for thinking outside the box, as their cognitive patterns are not always bound by traditional or linear thought processes. This can lead to innovative solutions and novel ideas.

5. **Emotional Sensitivity:** Many individuals with TS experience heightened emotional sensitivity, and this emotional richness can be channeled into creative expression. Their ability to connect deeply with their emotions and translate these feelings into their work can result in profoundly moving and relatable creative works.

6. **Compulsive Creative Processes:** In some cases, individuals with TS and OCTs may develop compulsive creative processes.

They might feel compelled to create art, music, or literature, which can lead to a prolific body of work and innovative approaches to their chosen creative outlets.

The relationship between Obsessive-Compulsive Traits and creativity in individuals with Tourette Syndrome is complex. While these traits may present certain advantages in creative processes, it's crucial to consider the individual's unique characteristics and experiences when examining the impact of OCTs on their creative endeavors.

Neuroimaging Studies

Neuroimaging studies have played a crucial role in shedding light on the relationship between Tourette Syndrome (TS) and creativity. These studies have provided valuable insights into the brain structures and functions associated with TS, which, in turn, have helped researchers understand how TS may influence cognitive processes related to creativity. Here's how neuroimaging studies contribute to our understanding of the TS-creativity relationship:

1. **Identification of Brain Abnormalities:** Neuroimaging studies, such as MRI and fMRI (functional magnetic resonance imaging), have identified certain

structural and functional brain differences in individuals with TS. One common finding is alterations in the basal ganglia and frontal cortex, which are areas associated with motor control and inhibitory processes. These alterations are thought to contribute to the motor and vocal tics characteristic of TS.

2. **Neurological Networks:** Research has shown that the brain networks involved in TS often extend beyond motor functions. The prefrontal cortex, for example, is also linked to higher-order cognitive functions like decision-making, planning, and creativity. Neuroimaging studies have revealed that some individuals with TS may have differences

in how these brain regions communicate or function, potentially influencing creative thinking.

3. **Inhibition and Creativity:** Creativity is a multifaceted cognitive process that can involve breaking away from conventional thinking and generating novel ideas. Studies have indicated that TS is associated with an imbalance in inhibitory control processes. TS individuals may struggle to suppress unwanted behaviors, like tics, but this same trait might also encourage the generation of unique and unconventional ideas, which is a hallmark of creativity.

4. **Personality Traits:** Some studies have shown that individuals with TS may exhibit certain personality traits, such as increased impulsivity and openness to experience. These traits can be conducive to creativity as they encourage risk-taking and a willingness to explore new ideas.

It's important to note that while neuroimaging studies provide valuable insights, the relationship between TS and creativity is complex and multifaceted. Not all individuals with TS will necessarily exhibit enhanced creativity, and creativity itself is influenced by a multitude of factors, including genetic predispositions, environmental influences, and personal experiences.

Neuroimaging studies have helped uncover the neurological basis of TS and how it might influence creativity. By examining the structural and functional differences in the brains of individuals with TS, researchers can better understand the neurological processes that may underlie creative thinking in some individuals with this condition.

The relationship between TS and creativity is a complex and evolving area of study. While historical cases hint at intriguing connections, contemporary research offers more grounded insights. It is essential to recognize that TS is a heterogeneous condition, and not all individuals with TS will demonstrate exceptional creative talents.

The TS-creativity connection underscores the intricate nature of the human brain, where neurological variations can simultaneously present challenges and unlock exceptional creative potential. Further research and exploration in this field are necessary to unravel the mysteries of this fascinating relationship.

Chapter 6

The Neurological Basis of Creativity in Tourette Syndrome

Creativity is a multifaceted and complex cognitive process that encompasses the generation of novel ideas, original thinking, and the ability to produce innovative solutions. The neurological basis of creativity in individuals with Tourette Syndrome (TS) is an intriguing and evolving area of research. In this chapter, we will explore the brain structure and function associated with creativity in TS and delve into the concept of neurodiversity as it relates to creative thinking.

Brain Structure and Function

Understanding the neurological basis of creativity in TS requires an examination of the brain structures and functions associated with both the condition and creative thinking:

1. **Basal Ganglia**: The basal ganglia, a group of nuclei deep within the brain, plays a critical role in the motor control circuits and is closely linked to TS. Aberrations in the basal ganglia are believed to contribute to the generation of tics. Interestingly, the basal ganglia is also involved in cognitive processes such as cognitive flexibility and procedural learning. Some researchers suggest that the same neurological circuits that lead to

tics may also enhance creative thinking, as they enable individuals to approach problems from various angles and develop unique solutions.

2. **Frontal Cortex:** The frontal cortex, particularly the prefrontal cortex, is associated with executive functions like working memory, decision-making, and divergent thinking—all of which are crucial for creative thought. TS can affect the connectivity and activity within the frontal cortex, potentially contributing to both the tics and creative capabilities observed in individuals with the condition.

3. **Neurotransmitters:** Aberrations in neurotransmitter systems, particularly dopamine, have been implicated in TS. Dopamine is involved in reward and motivation, and it has been associated with creative thinking. The complex interplay of dopamine and other neurotransmitters in TS may influence cognitive processes, including creativity.

Chapter 7

Nurturing Creativity in TS Individuals

Tourette Syndrome (TS) is a neurodevelopmental disorder that can present a unique set of challenges, but it's also associated with remarkable strengths, particularly in the realm of creativity. Nurturing creativity in individuals with TS involves providing support, understanding, and opportunities for self-expression. In this chapter, we will explore strategies for parents and educators to help foster creativity in TS individuals and promote their artistic pursuits.

Strategies for Parents and Educators

1. **Education and Awareness**: The first step in nurturing creativity in TS individuals is to educate oneself and others about the condition. Parents and educators should have a solid understanding of TS, its symptoms, and the potential challenges it poses. This knowledge can help reduce stigma and create a more inclusive environment.

2. **Individualized Support**: Recognize that each TS individual is unique. Tailor support and accommodations to their specific needs and strengths. This might involve personalized education plans, therapy, or modifications to the learning environment.

3. **Open Communication**: Maintain open and honest communication with TS individuals. Encourage them to share their experiences, challenges, and creative aspirations. Listening attentively and without judgment is crucial.

4. **Stress Management**: TS symptoms can worsen with stress and anxiety. Teach stress management techniques such as deep breathing exercises, mindfulness, or relaxation strategies to help individuals manage their tics and create a conducive environment for creativity.

5. **Encourage Self-Advocacy**: Empower TS individuals to advocate for themselves and their creative needs. Encourage them to express their preferences and

concerns in educational and artistic settings.

6. **Flexibility and Patience**: Understand that TS symptoms can be unpredictable. Be flexible in your approach, and exercise patience when tics or other challenges arise. This patience can create a safe space for creative expression.

7. **Collaboration with Therapists**: Collaborate with therapists, such as occupational therapists or behavioral specialists, to develop strategies that support creative activities. These professionals can provide valuable guidance on how to adapt creative pursuits to the individual's needs.

Fostering Self-Expression and Artistic Pursuits

1. **Artistic Outlets**: Encourage TS individuals to explore various artistic outlets, such as visual arts, music, writing, or performance arts. Provide access to resources and materials that align with their interests.

2. **Creative Workshops**: Consider enrolling TS individuals in creative workshops or classes that align with their passions. These structured environments can provide both skill development and opportunities for self-expression.

3. **Positive Reinforcement**: Recognize and celebrate their creative efforts and achievements. Positive reinforcement can boost self-esteem and motivation to

continue pursuing artistic endeavors.

4. **Creative Challenges**: Offer creative challenges or projects that encourage TS individuals to think outside the box. These challenges can stimulate innovation and problem-solving while harnessing their creative potential.

5. **Collaborative Opportunities**: Encourage collaboration with peers and mentors. Collaboration can provide a sense of community and opportunities for learning and growth in creative pursuits.

6. **Art Therapy**: Consider art therapy as a means of self-expression and emotional release. Art therapists can help individuals with TS explore their feelings and experiences through creative

processes.

7. **Promote Self-Expression**: Emphasize that the creative process is a form of self-expression and communication. Encourage TS individuals to convey their thoughts, emotions, and unique perspectives through their art.

8. **Patience with Creative Blocks**: Creative blocks are common for artists of all backgrounds. Teach TS individuals that creative challenges are part of the process and that patience and persistence can overcome them.

Nurturing creativity in individuals with Tourette Syndrome involves a multifaceted approach that includes understanding, support, and encouragement. Parents and educators play a vital role in creating an environment where TS individuals can freely express themselves, develop their creative talents, and overcome challenges on their artistic journeys. By fostering creativity, we not only empower individuals with TS but also enrich our understanding of the profound creative potential that resides within the human mind.

Chapter 8

Creative Outlets for TS Individuals

Fostering creativity in individuals with Tourette Syndrome (TS) can be a powerful means of self-expression and personal growth. Creative outlets provide opportunities for TS individuals to channel their unique perspectives, emotions, and experiences into various art forms. In this section, we will explore creative outlets for TS individuals, including the benefits of art therapy and other avenues such as music, writing, and more.

Art Therapy and Its Benefits

Art therapy is a valuable therapeutic approach that involves using creative processes to explore and express emotions, reduce stress, and enhance overall well-being. It can be particularly beneficial for individuals with TS. Here are some key benefits of art therapy:

1. **Emotional Expression**: Art therapy provides a safe and non-verbal space for TS individuals to express their emotions. Many TS individuals grapple with emotional challenges related to their condition, and art can serve as a means of release and self-expression.

2. **Stress Reduction**: Engaging in art can be a relaxing and stress-reducing experience. The act of creating art can divert attention away from tics and worries, offering a calming and meditative outlet.

3. **Enhanced Self-Esteem**: Creating art and witnessing one's artistic growth can boost self-esteem. TS individuals may gain a sense of achievement, helping to counteract any negative self-perceptions related to their tics.

4. **Coping and Self-Regulation**: Art therapy can teach individuals with TS valuable skills for coping with their symptoms and managing stress. It helps them develop self-regulation strategies and enhances

their ability to focus and relax.

5. **Improved Communication**: Art provides an alternative mode of communication for TS individuals who may struggle with verbal expression. Through their art, they can convey thoughts, feelings, and experiences that might be challenging to put into words.

6. **Community and Support**: Participating in art therapy sessions often creates a sense of community and shared experience. This social aspect can provide a support network for individuals with TS, promoting a sense of belonging.

Music, Writing, and Other Creative Avenues

1. **Music**: Music offers a powerful medium for creative expression. Individuals with TS may find solace and creative fulfillment in playing musical instruments, singing, or composing music. The rhythmic and repetitive nature of music can be particularly appealing to some with TS, as it can align with their tics and provide a structured outlet for expression.

2. **Writing**: Writing, including journaling, poetry, and storytelling, is an effective means of self-expression for TS individuals. It allows them to explore their thoughts and feelings and share

their unique perspectives with others.

3. **Visual Arts**: Painting, drawing, sculpture, and other visual arts provide a canvas for creative expression. The process of creating visual art can be both therapeutic and deeply rewarding, allowing individuals to communicate and reflect on their experiences.

4. **Drama and Performance Arts**: Drama, acting, and performance arts offer a platform for TS individuals to step into different roles and explore their emotions in a controlled and structured environment. The stage can be a place where tics can be channeled into creative characters and narratives.

5. **Dance and Movement:** For some individuals, dance and movement provide an avenue for self-expression and creativity. These activities can help promote physical well-being and improve self-confidence.

6. **Creative Writing Workshops and Art Classes:** Enrolling in creative writing workshops or art classes tailored to individuals with TS can offer structured guidance and a supportive community for artistic growth.

Creative outlets for TS individuals are not only avenues for artistic expression but also sources of therapeutic benefits and personal development. Art therapy, as well as various creative avenues like music, writing, and the visual and performing arts, provide unique and valuable opportunities for individuals with TS to harness their creativity and share their experiences with the world. These outlets empower TS individuals to thrive in their artistic pursuits while promoting overall well-being and self-expression.

Chapter 9

Support Systems and Resources

For individuals living with Tourette Syndrome (TS), having access to support systems and resources is essential in navigating the challenges and embracing the strengths associated with the condition. In this section, we will explore the various organizations and communities that offer support for TS individuals, as well as the therapeutic and educational resources available to help them and their families.

Organizations and Communities for TS Individuals

1. **Tourette Association of America (TAA):** TAA is a prominent nonprofit organization dedicated to providing support, information, and advocacy for individuals and families affected by TS. They offer resources, educational materials, support groups, and events to raise awareness and provide a sense of community.

2. **Tourette Syndrome Foundation of Canada:** This Canadian organization offers similar support, resources, and advocacy for individuals and families in Canada dealing with TS.

3. **Tourettes Action (UK)**: Tourettes Action is a leading support organization in the United Kingdom, offering information, support, and resources for individuals with TS and their families.

4. **Local Support Groups**: Many regions have local TS support groups that provide a sense of community, opportunities for families to connect, and a platform for individuals to share their experiences.

5. **Online Communities**: Online platforms, including forums, social media groups, and websites, provide valuable resources and opportunities for TS individuals to connect with others worldwide. These platforms can be particularly helpful for individuals who may face geographic

limitations in accessing support.

Therapeutic and Educational Resources

1. **Art Therapy:** Art therapy can be a powerful tool for individuals with TS to express themselves and manage their symptoms. Certified art therapists can help individuals explore their emotions and challenges through art-making.

2. **Music Therapy:** Music therapy is a therapeutic approach that uses music as a medium for emotional expression and stress reduction. It can be particularly beneficial for individuals with TS who are drawn to music and rhythm.

3. **Cognitive-Behavioral Therapy (CBT):** CBT is a well-established therapeutic approach that can help individuals

manage the emotional and psychological aspects of TS. It provides coping strategies to address tics, anxiety, and related challenges.

4. **Medication Management:** Individuals with TS may consider medical interventions to manage their symptoms. Consulting a healthcare professional, such as a neurologist or psychiatrist, is crucial in determining the appropriate medications, if needed, and monitoring their effects.

5. **Educational Resources:** Educational resources, such as books, articles, and online courses, offer valuable information on TS, its symptoms, and strategies for managing the condition. These resources

can be especially beneficial for parents, teachers, and individuals looking to better understand TS.

6. **Occupational Therapy**: Occupational therapists can assist individuals with TS in developing strategies to improve their ability to manage daily tasks and work-related challenges. This therapy can enhance independence and self-sufficiency.

7. **Speech and Language Therapy**: For individuals with TS who experience vocal tics, speech and language therapy can help improve communication and manage tic-related challenges.

8. **Parent Training Programs:** These programs provide parents with skills and strategies for effectively supporting their children with TS. They can address issues related to managing tics, social challenges, and educational needs.

9. **Legal and Educational Advocacy**: Legal and educational resources can be invaluable in securing appropriate accommodations and support in school and workplace settings. Legal experts or advocacy organizations can provide guidance in this regard.

Accessing these support systems and resources is crucial in enhancing the quality of life for individuals with TS and their families. They offer practical strategies for managing symptoms, a sense of belonging through community and advocacy organizations, and therapeutic interventions that cater to the unique challenges and strengths associated with Tourette Syndrome.

Chapter 10

Overcoming Stigma and Misconceptions

Tourette Syndrome (TS) is a neurodevelopmental condition characterized by involuntary motor and vocal tics. Unfortunately, TS has often been shrouded in stigma and misconceptions, leading to social challenges for individuals living with the condition. In this chapter, we will explore strategies to overcome stigma and misconceptions surrounding TS, emphasizing the importance of raising awareness, reducing stereotypes, and promoting inclusivity and acceptance.

Raising Awareness and Reducing Stereotypes

Education Initiatives: Educational programs targeting schools, communities, and the general public are crucial in raising awareness about TS. These initiatives should provide accurate information about the condition, its symptoms, and its impact on individuals and families.

Media Representation: Encourage responsible and accurate portrayals of TS in media and popular culture. Misrepresentation or caricatured depictions in movies, TV shows, and books can perpetuate stereotypes and create misunderstanding.

TS Advocacy Organizations: Support organizations and advocacy groups dedicated to TS awareness and support. These organizations often engage in public awareness campaigns and provide resources for individuals and families affected by TS.

Celebrities and Role Models: Promote positive role models who have TS and have achieved success in various fields. Their stories can inspire others and challenge stereotypes.

Community Workshops and Seminars: Organize workshops, seminars, and public talks to provide opportunities for people to learn more about TS. Personal stories and expert presentations can dispel myths and encourage open dialogue.

Online Resources: Make reliable and accessible online resources available for individuals seeking information about TS. Encourage the creation of online communities where people can share their experiences and support one another.

Promoting Inclusivity and Acceptance

School Inclusivity: Ensure that schools create inclusive environments for students with TS. This may involve educating teachers, classmates, and school staff about the condition and implementing accommodations to support students with TS in their academic pursuits.

Accommodations and support for students with Tourette Syndrome (TS) can help create an inclusive and conducive learning environment. Here are some accommodations that can be beneficial for students with TS:

1. **Educational Plan:** Develop an Individualized Education Plan (IEP) or a 504 Plan to outline specific accommodations and support services tailored to the student's needs.

2. **Quiet and Distraction-Free Space:** Provide a quiet, distraction-free area where the student can work or take breaks when needed to reduce stress and manage tics.

3. **Extended Time for Tests:** Allow extra time for completing tests and assignments, as tics may slow down the student's work pace.

4. **Alternative Testing Arrangements:** Offer a separate room for testing to minimize the impact of tics on the student's performance and to reduce anxiety.

5. **Breaks and Movement:** Allow for short breaks during class to let the student release tics, stretch, or walk around. Provide opportunities for physical activity to help manage tics and restlessness.

6. **Note-Taking Assistance:** Assign a peer note-taker or provide access to class notes in advance to assist the student in

case tics affect their ability to write or focus.

7.   **Flexible Seating:** Allow the student to sit where they are most comfortable in the classroom, so they can better manage their tics without disruption.

8.   **Use of Technology:** Provide assistive technology, such as speech-to-text software, to aid in written assignments and tests.

9.   **Communication with Peers:** Educate classmates and promote understanding to reduce potential stigma and bullying. Encourage students to be supportive and accepting.

10. **Emotional Support:** Offer access to a school counselor or mental health professional to help the student manage any emotional or social challenges that may arise.

11. **Structured Routines:** Establish predictable routines and schedules, which can help students with TS manage anxiety and minimize tics triggered by uncertainty.

12. **Frequent Check-Ins:** Regularly check in with the student to ensure they are coping well and to address any concerns or changes in their needs.

13. **Educational Materials:** Use visual aids and multisensory materials to enhance learning and engage the student more

effectively.

14. **Positive Reinforcement:** Implement a system of positive reinforcement and praise to motivate and boost the student's confidence.

15. **Flexibility on Assignments:** Allow the student flexibility in how they complete assignments. For example, they might submit video presentations or oral reports instead of written ones.

16. **Peer Awareness Programs:** Consider organizing peer awareness programs or presentations about TS to foster understanding and reduce stigma.

17. **Training for Educators:** Provide training for teachers and school staff about TS, its manifestations, and

strategies for supporting students with the condition.

18. **Regular Meetings:** Schedule regular meetings with parents, teachers, and the student to assess progress, adapt accommodations, and ensure consistent support.

19. **Sensory-Friendly Classroom:** Create a sensory-friendly classroom environment with controlled lighting and noise, if necessary, to reduce sensory triggers.

20. **Promote Self-Advocacy:** Encourage the student to develop self-advocacy skills, helping them communicate their needs to teachers and peers.

Remember that accommodations should be tailored to the specific needs of each student with TS, as the condition can vary widely in its presentation. Collaborative efforts between teachers, parents, and support professionals are essential to provide the most effective support and ensure a successful educational experience for the student.

Workplace Accommodations: Encourage workplaces to provide accommodations for employees with TS. These may include flexible work hours, remote work options, or understanding supervisors and colleagues who are aware of the condition.

Anti-Bullying Initiatives: Develop and support anti-bullying programs in schools and communities. TS individuals are often targets of teasing and bullying due to their tics, and such initiatives can help create safer spaces.

Mental Health Support: Recognize the psychological impact of living with TS and provide access to mental health support services. This support can be crucial for both individuals with TS and their families.

Health support services for people with Tourette Syndrome (TS) are essential to ensure they receive comprehensive care, manage their symptoms effectively, and lead fulfilling lives. Here are some key health support services available for individuals with TS:

1. **Medical Assessment and Diagnosis:** A healthcare provider, typically a neurologist or a specialist in movement disorders, can provide an accurate diagnosis of TS. They may also rule out other conditions that could be causing tic-like symptoms.

2. **Medication Management:** In cases where tics are severe and significantly impact the individual's quality of life, medication may be prescribed. Common medications for TS include antipsychotics and alpha-2 adrenergic agonists. These should be carefully monitored by a healthcare provider.

3. **Behavioral Therapies:** Behavioral therapies like Comprehensive Behavioral Intervention for Tics (CBIT) or Habit Reversal Training (HRT) can help individuals manage and reduce tic symptoms. A therapist or trained specialist typically conducts these therapies.

4. **Counseling and Psychotherapy:** Individuals with TS may experience anxiety, depression, or other psychological challenges. Mental health professionals can provide therapy and support to address these issues.

5. **Support Groups:** Joining TS support groups or community organizations can offer valuable emotional support, shared

experiences, and practical advice from others facing similar challenges.

6. **Health and Wellness Promotion:** Encourage a healthy lifestyle that includes regular exercise, a balanced diet, and adequate sleep. These factors can positively impact the severity of tics and overall well-being.

7. **Assistive Technologies:** Assistive technologies like speech recognition software can help individuals with TS overcome challenges associated with tics. It's crucial for individuals with TS to have a supportive healthcare team and access to a range of health support services that can address the complex and varied needs associated with the condition. The

combination of medical treatment, behavioral therapies, counseling, and educational support can significantly improve the quality of life for individuals with Tourette Syndrome.

Peer Support Groups: Establish or support peer support groups for individuals with TS. These groups can provide a sense of belonging, as members share common experiences and challenges.

Advocacy and Legislation: Advocate for legislation that protects the rights of individuals with TS and ensures that they have equal access to education, employment, and public services.

Community Engagement: Encourage TS individuals to engage with their communities and participate in social and artistic activities. This not only promotes acceptance but also helps individuals with TS feel more integrated and valued.

In conclusion, overcoming stigma and misconceptions surrounding Tourette Syndrome is a vital step in promoting a more inclusive and accepting society. Raising awareness through education, advocating for legislative protections, and providing resources for individuals and families can help reduce stereotypes and create a more empathetic and supportive environment for those living with TS. By fostering understanding and acceptance, we can ensure that individuals with TS can fully participate in all aspects of life, free from the burden of societal prejudice.

Chapter 11

The Future of TS Research and Creativity

As we look ahead, the field of Tourette Syndrome (TS) research continues to evolve, offering promising avenues for understanding the condition and harnessing the creative potential of TS individuals. In this section, we will explore ongoing studies, potential breakthroughs, and the importance of embracing the gifts of TS individuals.

Ongoing Studies and Potential Breakthroughs

1. **Genetic Research**: Ongoing genetic research is shedding light on the underlying causes of TS. Identifying specific genetic markers associated with TS could lead to more accurate diagnostic methods and potential targeted treatments.

2. **Neuroimaging**: Advancements in neuroimaging techniques, such as functional magnetic resonance imaging (fMRI), are enabling researchers to study the brain activity of individuals with TS. This research can provide insights into the neural mechanisms underlying tics and creativity.

3. **Behavioral Therapies:** Research into behavioral therapies and interventions is continually refining our understanding of effective treatments for TS. Cognitive-behavioral therapy (CBT), habit reversal therapy, and exposure and response prevention (ERP) are among the approaches showing promise in managing TS symptoms.

4. **Medication Development:** Pharmaceutical research continues to explore new medications and treatment options for TS. These developments aim to improve symptom management with fewer side effects.

5. **Neurodiversity Perspective**: The concept of neurodiversity is gaining traction in the field of TS research. Embracing the neurodiversity perspective acknowledges that TS, like other neurodevelopmental conditions, represents a unique way of thinking and experiencing the world. This shift in perspective fosters inclusivity and appreciation of TS individuals' creative talents.

6. **Personalized Medicine**: As research advances, personalized medicine approaches are becoming more feasible. Tailoring treatments and interventions to the specific needs and strengths of TS individuals holds the potential for more effective symptom management and

improved quality of life.

Embracing the Gifts of TS Individuals

1. **Creative Potential**: As the link between TS and creativity becomes more evident, society should continue to embrace and celebrate the creative potential of TS individuals. This recognition can empower them to pursue careers in various creative fields.

2. **Advocacy and Awareness**: Advocacy efforts should continue to promote awareness and understanding of TS. Emphasizing the strengths and unique perspectives of TS individuals can challenge stereotypes and reduce stigma.

3. **Education and Inclusivity**: Schools and workplaces can further promote inclusivity and accommodate the needs of TS individuals. By understanding the condition and its implications, educational and professional institutions can create environments that foster the success of TS individuals.

4. **Support Systems**: Families, support organizations, and communities should provide the necessary support and resources to help TS individuals thrive. Encouraging self-advocacy, self-expression, and mental health support can make a significant difference in their well-being.

5. **Inspiration and Role Models:** TS individuals who have achieved success in their respective fields can serve as inspirational role models. Their stories can motivate others to embrace their unique talents and pursue their passions, regardless of their condition.

In conclusion, the future of TS research holds great promise for understanding and managing the condition more effectively. It also provides an opportunity to shift societal attitudes and embrace the creative potential of TS individuals. By supporting ongoing research, promoting inclusivity, and celebrating the talents and accomplishments of TS individuals, we can work towards a future where individuals with TS are valued for their unique perspectives and contributions to the world.

Conclusion

Tourette Syndrome (TS) is a complex and often misunderstood neurodevelopmental condition that has both its challenges and unique strengths. In this exploration, we've delved into the multifaceted world of TS, its connection to creativity, and the support systems that can help individuals with TS thrive. As we conclude, let's celebrate the unique gifts of TS individuals and look ahead to a more inclusive and creative world.

TS individuals often possess remarkable creative talents. The condition's link to enhanced cognitive flexibility, divergent thinking, and intense focus can be harnessed in various artistic and innovative endeavors.

Living with TS requires a high level of resilience. Individuals with TS often face societal stigma, social challenges, and the need to manage their symptoms daily. Their resilience is a testament to their inner strength. TS individuals can be highly empathetic, as they understand the challenges of navigating a world that doesn't always accommodate their needs. This empathy can foster a deep connection with others facing similar challenges. Many TS individuals are passionate advocates, working to raise awareness, reduce stigma, and promote understanding of the condition. Their advocacy efforts help shape a more inclusive society.

The concept of neurodiversity is gaining traction and reshaping the way society views conditions like TS. Embracing neurodiversity acknowledges that different neurological variations are valuable and contribute to the richness of the human experience. Communities, families, schools, and workplaces can create supportive environments that cater to the needs and strengths of TS individuals. By offering understanding, accommodations, and encouragement, we can help TS individuals reach their full potential.

Tourette Syndrome is more than just a set of symptoms; it's a condition that embodies the remarkable potential of the human mind. By celebrating the unique gifts of TS individuals and fostering a more inclusive and creative world, we can ensure that everyone, regardless of their neurological diversity, has the opportunity to thrive and contribute to the betterment of society. Embracing diversity in all its forms is not just a moral imperative but also a path to a more vibrant, innovative, and empathetic world.

www.ingramcontent.com/pod-product-compliance
Lightning Source LLC
Chambersburg PA
CBHW050823260726
48660CB00004B/1570